PEPPERMINT OIL

A Comprehensive Guide to its Remarkable Health Benefits and Natural Remedies By Unlocking the Power of Peppermint Oil

SAMANTHA ZYLAR

Contents

CHAPTER ONE 6

Overview 6

The Universe Of Mint Oil 6

Historische Bedeutung: 7

Creation And Formulation: 8

Uses In Practice And Therapy: ...9

Fragrant Origins 11

Aromatic Origins: 11

A Synopsis Of Peppermint's History: 12

The History And Culture Of Peppermint: 13

This Is A Condensed Explanation Of The Distillation Procedure: 15

Ingredients In Peppermint Oil 18

The Science Of Peppermint Oil: 19

How Ingredients Affect Fragrance And Advantages: 21

CHAPTER TWO 26

The Aroma Of Wellbeing 26

Peppermint Oil And Aromatherapy 26

Essential Oils And Peppermint Oil 27

The Effects Of Peppermint Oil On Emotions And Mood 29

Practical Applications For Peppermint Aromatherapy.......31

Peppermint Oil's Health And Healing Properties 34

The Therapeutic Aspects Of Peppermint Oil: 35

Reducing Pain And Aches:......36

Digestive Health: Treating Nausea And Indigestion: 38

Peppermint Oil For Personal Care And Beauty 40

1. Peppermint Oil For Cosmetic Uses: 41

2. Applying Peppermint Oil To Hair Care: 42

3. Natural Treatments For Typical Skin And Hair Problems: 44

4. Handcrafted Cosmetics:......45

CHAPTER THREE 48

Adventures In Cooking With Peppermint....................................48

Mint Leaves In The Kitchen....49

From Desserts To Drinks.........50

The Uses Of Peppermint Oil In Cooking 52

Using Peppermint Oil In Daily Life 54

1. Natural Solutions For Pest Control With Peppermint Oil: .55

2. Peppermint For Cleaning And Freshening: 57

3. Peppermint Oil In Dental Care: 59

Warnings And Points To Take 61

Take These Safety Measures Before Using Peppermint Oil: .62

Sensitive Groups, Allergies, And Interactions: 64

Dose:..65

Avoids: 67

Conclusion...................................68

CHAPTER ONE

Overview

The Universe Of Mint Oil

For millennia, people all around the world have been drawn to and appreciated the engaging and adaptable properties of peppermint oil.

Peppermint oil is widely used in many different businesses, customs, and civilizations due to its energizing qualities, pleasant aroma, and numerous uses. This overview explores the intriguing world of peppermint oil, including information on its composition, history, manufacturing process, and several practical and medicinal applications.

Historische Bedeutung:

Menth piperita, the scientific name for peppermint, has a long and illustrious history that dates back to ancient times. Because of its therapeutic qualities, it was highly valued in the traditional medicine of many cultures, including the Greeks, Romans, and Egyptians.

Greek mythology and ancient Egyptian medical literature both make reference to the usage of peppermint oil. This long history implies that people have been drawn to peppermint oil for thousands of years.

Creation And Formulation:

The usual methods for obtaining peppermint oil is to steam distill the leaves and flowering tops of the peppermint plant. Menthol is one of the most noticeable chemical constituents in the oil's composition. Menthol is a common ingredient in many products, such as over-the-counter medicines, cosmetics, and dental care products.

It also provides peppermint oil with its distinctive cooling effect.

Menthone, menthofuran, and a variety of other chemical compounds are also included in peppermint oil's makeup, which adds to its distinct aroma and medicinal benefits.

Uses In Practice And Therapy:

Because of its many useful applications, peppermint oil is a common household staple due to its versatility. It is often used in aromatherapy and as an ingredient in scented candles, diffusers, and room sprays due to its well-known, energizing, and refreshing perfume. Beyond a pleasant aroma, peppermint oil has many medicinal uses. It is well renowned for its capacity to ease headaches and tension, ease intestinal discomfort, and promote respiratory health. Because of the oil's calming and relaxing qualities, cosmetic products and muscle relief remedies now contain it.

The benefits of peppermint oil go beyond personal hygiene. In the culinary arts, it is used to improve the flavor of a variety of foods and drinks. In the agricultural industry, the oil is also used as a natural insecticide to keep pests from harming crops.

We will examine each of these aspects as we go deeper into the realm of peppermint oil, from its historical significance to its many contemporary applications. We will explore the mysteries surrounding this exceptional oil and recognize its lasting appeal across a range of societies, sectors, and daily existence. Come along on this olfactory journey into the fascinating history, intriguing present, and exciting future of peppermint oil.

Fragrant Origins

Aromatic Origins:

Peppermint oil is a versatile essential oil that has captivated people's senses for generations with its energizing and refreshing perfume. Its path from antiquity to contemporary applications is evidence of its lasting appeal and wide range of applications. We explore the fragrant origins, lengthy history, and complex procedures that go into making peppermint oil in this investigation.

A Synopsis Of Peppermint's History:

Peppermint was highly valued for its culinary and medicinal properties in ancient civilizations. The Egyptians, Greeks, and Romans employed it, and its origins may be found in Europe and Asia. Peppermint was used for its medicinal benefits and even made its way into pharaohs' tombs in ancient

Egypt, demonstrating its importance at the time. On the other hand, peppermint was used in food and drink by the Greeks and Romans, who understood its culinary benefits.

The History And Culture Of Peppermint:

Peppermint (Mentha piperita) is a hybrid mint that is said to have originated from a cross between spearmint (Mentha spicata) and watermint (Mentha aquatica). It is well-known for growing quickly, being hardy, and spreading easily by subterranean rhizomes. Since ancient times, peppermint plants have been grown for centuries in locations with mild climates, including Europe, the Middle East, and Asia.

For peppermint plants to be vigorous and fragrant, they need well-drained soil, lots of sunlight, and frequent trimming. Crushed leaves exude the unique peppermint aroma that has come to be associated with the plant. Peppermint plants require close attention to achieve maximum oil production, thus cultivating them is a laborious procedure.

The powerful and highly sought-after peppermint oil is made from the leaves of the peppermint plant through a process called distillation and extraction. Steam distillation is the most widely used extraction technique, which uses steam pressure to extract the essential oil from plant material.

This Is A Condensed Explanation Of The Distillation Procedure:

1. Harvesting: When the oil content of mature peppermint plants reaches its maximum, usually during the flowering period, they are harvested.

2. Distillation: Steam distillation involves passing steam through a container containing crushed plant material in order to extract the leaves that have been gathered. The essential

oil is released when the leaves' oil sacs burst due to the steam.

3. Condensation: The essential oil is extracted from the water and other plant components by condensing the steam, which is now transporting the oil, back into a liquid condition.

4. Gathering: The gathered liquid undergoes additional separation, with the essential oil ascending to the top as a result of its reduced density. This oil is commonly referred to as peppermint oil.

5. Bottling: To maintain its strength and fragrance, the last of the peppermint oil is meticulously

bottled, sealed, and kept in a cold, dark area.

The voyage of peppermint oil from ancient civilizations to modern manufacturing processes has allowed its aromatic legacy to persist. Peppermint oil is appreciated for its varied applications, from aromatherapy to culinary pleasures. Regardless of your preference for its calming aroma, digestive advantages, or a taste boost in your preferred recipe, peppermint oil persistently provides a fragrant entryway to an infinite array of opportunities.

Ingredients In Peppermint Oil

Made from the leaves of the peppermint plant (Mentha × piperita), peppermint oil is well known for both its stimulating scent and a host of possible health advantages. The intricate chemical makeup of peppermint oil is responsible for its unique qualities. We will examine the chemistry of peppermint oil in this talk, including its main ingredients—menthol, menthone, and other compounds—and how they affect the oil's scent and related health benefits.

The Science Of Peppermint Oil:

A wide variety of chemical components are present in peppermint oil, and each one contributes to its distinct qualities. The following are the main ingredients of peppermint oil:

1. The most noticeable and well-known ingredient in peppermint oil is menthol. When administered topically or breathed, it gives off a distinctive chilly feeling. Due to its analgesic qualities, menthol is frequently included as a component in topical pain treatment solutions.

2. Menthone: Menthone is another important ingredient that gives peppermint oil its minty scent. It may also have medicinal uses, such as promoting better digestion and relieving headaches.

3. Menthyl Acetate: This substance gives the scent of the oil a fruity, sweet undertone. It is frequently used in aromatherapy for relaxation because of its calming qualities.

4. 1,8-Cineole, also known as eucalyptol, is a small yet important component of peppermint oil. It adds to the earthy, slightly woodsy aspects of the oil and has been researched for

possible anti-inflammatory and respiratory properties.

5. Limonene: A common terpene present in many essential oils, limonene gives peppermint oil its zesty scent. It is well-recognized for having possible mood-boosting and antioxidant qualities.

How Ingredients Affect Fragrance And Advantages:

The way the molecules in peppermint oil work together harmoniously gives it its unique scent. Peppermint oil is a popular choice in aromatherapy because of its exhilarating and refreshing smell, which is primarily imparted by menthol and menthone.

The ingredients in peppermint oil have several possible advantages in addition to its scent.

• Aromatherapy: The scent of peppermint oil helps relieve tension and headaches, boost alertness, and lessen mental weariness. The body and mind may feel revitalized by inhaling the oil.

• Digestive Health: By calming the gastrointestinal tract's muscles, menthone and other chemicals in peppermint oil may help with digestion. It is frequently used to relieve bloating, gas, and stomach symptoms.

• Topical Uses: Peppermint oil is a popular option for topical treatments due to the menthol's cooling effect. It can ease tension, ease tight muscles, and even soothe minor skin irritations.

• Respiratory Health: By opening airways and relieving congestion, eucalyptol and other chemicals may assist in improving respiratory health. Those who have allergies or colds would especially benefit from this.

In summary, the chemistry of peppermint oil reveals a rich combination of chemicals that support both its various therapeutic uses and reviving scent. Together, menthol, menthone, and other ingredients make peppermint oil a widely used and adaptable essential oil for wellness, skincare, and aromatherapy.

CHAPTER TWO

The Aroma Of Wellbeing

Peppermint Oil And Aromatherapy

Aromatherapy is a natural and holistic approach to health that has gained popularity in recent years. It involves using essential oils to improve both physical and psychological well-being.

With so many uses, peppermint oil is one of the most beneficial and adaptable essential oils on the market. This article delves into the fascinating realm of peppermint oil, examining its effects on emotions and mood as well as its useful applications in aromatherapy.

Essential Oils And Peppermint Oil

The power of smell to influence our emotions, mental states, and physical health is harnessed by aromatherapy. The principal instruments in aromatherapy are essential oils, which are extracted from different types of plants.

Of these, peppermint oil is highly regarded for its distinct qualities. This oil is derived from the leaves of the Mentha × piperita peppermint plant and has a strong menthol content that gives it a revitalizing and cool smell.

Because peppermint oil stimulates and awakens the senses, it is frequently used in aromatherapy. It releases a fresh, minty scent when diffused into the atmosphere, which can improve energy, encourage mental clarity, and even lessen the symptoms of some illnesses, such as headaches and lung congestion.

Peppermint is a great option for anyone in need of a mental boost because the scent of the plant may make you feel awake and fresh.

The Effects Of Peppermint Oil On Emotions And Mood

The aroma of peppermint oil has a strong effect on feelings and mood. Due to its well-known ability to elevate mood, this essential oil is a useful tool for stress, anxiety, and mood swing management. The following are a few ways that peppermint oil might affect feelings:

1. Stress Reduction: By encouraging calmness and relaxation, peppermint oil inhalation helps lessen tension and anxiety. It is an excellent natural stress reliever that may be applied in

both home and professional environments.

2. Mental Clarity: The stimulating aroma of peppermint oil helps enhance focus and mental clarity. This makes it a great option for anyone who needs to focus on their work or study efficiently.

3. Emotional Balance: Peppermint oil is a useful tool for people who are experiencing emotional turbulence or low energy levels because it may help regulate mood swings and raise one's spirits.

4. Headache Relief: Because peppermint oil has calming, cooling qualities, aromatherapy using it can

help relieve headaches and migraines. It can be diffused for inhalation or applied topically to the temples.

Practical Applications For Peppermint Aromatherapy

The practical applications of peppermint oil in aromatherapy are numerous due to its versatility. You can include peppermint oil in the following ways as part of your regular wellness routine:

1. Diffusion: To create a positive and revitalizing ambiance in your home or business, add a few drops of

peppermint oil to an essential oil diffuser.

2. Topical Application: To feel the calming and mood-enhancing benefits of peppermint oil, dilute it with a carrier oil (such as jojoba or coconut oil) and apply it to the back of the neck or pulse points.

3. Inhalation: For a rapid energy boost or stress reduction during the day, inhale straight from the bottle or add a few drops to a tissue.

4. Bath Soak: Infuse your bathwater with a few drops of peppermint oil to enhance your bathing experience. You'll feel rejuvenated and at ease thanks to the perfume and steam.

5. Massage Oil: To make a reviving massage oil that is ideal for relieving aching muscles and energizing the body, blend peppermint oil with a carrier oil.

In summary, peppermint oil has a revitalizing and refreshing aroma, is a key component of aromatherapy, and has a favorable effect on mood, feelings, and general well-being. Adding peppermint oil to your wellness arsenal can be beneficial for relieving stress, improving mental clarity, or just enjoying a refreshing aroma. When using essential oils, especially peppermint, always remember to use caution and adhere to the specified dilution and safety requirements.

Peppermint Oil's Health And Healing Properties

For generations, people have used peppermint oil, which is made from the leaves of the peppermint plant (Mentha × piperita), as a natural cure for a variety of health problems.

Due to its many medical uses, it is a well-liked option for treating a variety of illnesses. In this piece, we'll examine the medicinal uses of peppermint oil, emphasizing how it can help with aches and pains and how it can support digestive health by easing nausea and indigestion.

The Therapeutic Aspects Of Peppermint Oil:

1. Benefits of Peppermint Oil: Peppermint oil is well-known for its analgesic and anti-inflammatory qualities. It has ingredients like menthol that have anti-inflammatory and pain-relieving properties. Applying peppermint oil topically can help relieve headaches, aches in the muscles, and pain in the joints. Sore spots may feel relieved and relaxed by its cooling effect.

2. The Cooling Effect of Menthol: When applied topically, menthol, the main active ingredient in peppermint oil, produces a cooling effect. This feeling is very helpful for easing the discomfort brought on by headaches, migraines, and even sunburns since it can help dull the pain and bring comfort.

Reducing Pain And Aches:

There are several ways to utilize peppermint oil to ease aches and pains:

• Topical Application: Apply a few drops of peppermint oil, diluted with a carrier oil (such as almond or coconut oil), to the area that is afflicted. Apply the oil gently to your skin for a calming, cooling effect.

• Aromatherapy: One great way to treat headaches brought on by stress is to diffuse peppermint oil into the air. This will help you relax and release tension from your muscles.

• Bath Soak: A warm bath enhanced with a few drops of peppermint oil helps ease tight muscles and encourage relaxation.

Digestive Health: Treating Nausea And Indigestion:

The benefits of peppermint oil for digestion are well-known:

• Relieving Indigestion: Peppermint oil has the ability to ease the gastrointestinal tract's tense muscles, which may lessen indigestion's symptoms including bloating and pain. To help with digestion, you can drink peppermint tea or take enteric-coated peppermint oil capsules.

• Assisting with Nausea: Studies have shown that the aroma of peppermint helps with motion sickness and nausea. To aid with nausea management, you can inhale the aroma of peppermint oil or sip peppermint tea.

• Irritable Bowel Syndrome (IBS): Because enteric-coated peppermint oil capsules release the oil in the intestines, where it is most helpful, some IBS sufferers experience relief from symptoms including gas and stomach pain.

Because of its therapeutic qualities, peppermint oil is a useful natural medicine for treating pains and easing stomach issues. Peppermint oil's adaptability and calming properties can be a welcome addition to your health and healing toolkit, whether you want to reduce muscle stiffness, soothe indigestion, or fight nausea. But, it's crucial to use peppermint oil carefully. Make sure you adhere to the suggested dilution requirements and see a doctor if you have any particular medical conditions or concerns.

Peppermint Oil For Personal Care And Beauty

Because of its many advantages for skincare and haircare, peppermint oil is a multipurpose essential oil that has grown in popularity in the personal care and beauty sector. This essential oil, which is extracted from the leaves of the peppermint plant (Mentha piperita), is a popular component of many cosmetic products due to its energizing and refreshing aroma. Here are some uses for peppermint oil in cosmetics and personal hygiene:

1. Peppermint Oil For Cosmetic Uses:

• Acne Treatment: Peppermint oil works well to treat acne since it has antibacterial and anti-inflammatory qualities. It can be administered topically to lessen the redness and inflammation brought on by acne when diluted with a carrier oil (such as coconut or jojoba oil).

• Cooling feeling: The skin feels refreshed and soothed by the cooling feeling of peppermint oil. Invigorating effects can be achieved by mixing it with face mists and toners, particularly in hot weather.

• Diminishing Redness: The oil's anti-inflammatory qualities help to lessen redness brought on by rosacea or other skin irritations.

2. Applying Peppermint Oil To Hair Care:

• Health of the Scalp: Using peppermint oil can help maintain a healthy scalp. Because of its menthol concentration, which aids in blood circulation, it may encourage hair growth and lessen dandruff.

• Hair Growth: Some people include peppermint oil in their regimen to promote hair growth. It is frequently mixed with carrier oil for scalp massages or added to shampoos and conditioners.

• Refreshing Hair: Peppermint oil is included in hair products because of its energizing scent, which makes showers feel revitalizing and energizing.

3. Natural Treatments For Typical Skin And Hair Problems:

• Sunburn Relief: Sunburned skin may feel better because of peppermint oil's cooling properties. Topical application of diluted mixture with aloe vera gel or carrier oil helps alleviate pain and reduce inflammation.

• Itchy Scalp: The calming qualities of peppermint oil help to relieve itchy scalp irritation. It can be used to ease discomfort by combining it with a carrier oil and gently massaging the scalp.

• Strengthening of Hair: Combining peppermint oil with other essential oils, such as lavender and rosemary, can help create healthier, stronger hair.

4. Handcrafted Cosmetics:

• For individuals who would rather create their own beauty products, peppermint oil is a popular option. This essential oil can be used to make homemade facial masks, scrubs, lip balms, and hair treatments.

• Because of its adaptability, you can customize items to meet your unique hair and skincare requirements.

• Natural and organic ingredients are given priority in DIY beauty products using peppermint oil, which makes them a good choice for people who want chemical-free alternatives.

Before applying it to the skin or hair, always dilute it with carrier oil because it can be rather strong and irritating if applied undiluted. Additionally, before using products containing peppermint oil on their face or body, people with sensitive skin should perform a patch test. Peppermint oil may be a naturally refreshing addition to your beauty and personal care routine when used with consideration.

CHAPTER THREE

Adventures In Cooking
With Peppermint

For generations, peppermint has been a cherished herb in culinary traditions due to its revitalizing and refreshing taste. Its unique flavor and scent make it a flexible component that may be used to prepare a variety of foods, from drinks to sweets. Adding peppermint oil to your food is a fun and interesting way to give it a gourmet touch. Come along for a taste trip as we explore the many culinary applications of peppermint oil.

Mint Leaves In The Kitchen

The culinary world has long loved peppermint, a perennial herb noted for its vivid green leaves and strong menthol flavor.

Peppermint leaves, whether fresh or dried, add a crisp flavor to a variety of meals.

But the real culinary magic is found in peppermint oil, which provides concentrated peppermint flavor and is a favorite with home cooks and chefs alike.

From Desserts To Drinks

1. Drinks Infused with Peppermint: Peppermint oil is a key component in making cool drinks. For a refreshing hit of răcor, try a few drops in your mojito, iced tea, or lemonade. A just drop of peppermint oil can turn an ordinary glass of water into a refreshing concoction. Try it in smoothies to create a delicious blend of refreshing mint and fruits.

2. Tasty Mains: The distinct flavor of peppermint oil also enhances savory foods. Use it to marinate lamb and poultry or to make a tangy salad dressing. The zesty taste of

peppermint oil complements Mediterranean and Middle Eastern foods remarkably well, giving meals like tabbouleh or tzatziki a revitalizing edge.

3. Delicious Desserts: When it comes to desserts, peppermint oil really shines. You may make brownies, cakes, and cookies with peppermint flavoring. A dash of peppermint oil makes classic chocolate-mint combos even more appealing. Taste it in your homemade truffles or ice cream to enhance the decadent experience.

4. Refreshing Cocktails: Peppermint oil is a must-have for mixologists. Make your own artisanal cocktails,

including a peppermint patty cocktail, mint juleps, or martinis. Peppermint oil's vivid flavor and perfume can make your beverages stand out at any party.

The Uses Of Peppermint Oil In Cooking

A culinary treasure, peppermint oil offers the following advantages in the kitchen:

1. Concentration of Flavor: Peppermint oil has a highly concentrated herb flavor, thus a small amount goes a long way. It is hence an effective flavoring agent.

2. Long Shelf Life: Peppermint oil has a long shelf life, so you may enjoy its delicious flavor all year round, unlike fresh peppermint leaves.

3. Precise Control: You can create the right degree of peppermint flavor in your dishes by precisely controlling the amount of oil.

4. Versatility: Peppermint oil can be adjusted to meet your culinary demands, whether you're looking to add a strong blast of freshness or a subtle hint of mint.

In conclusion, the distinct and reviving flavor of peppermint oil elevates food to a whole new level, opening up a world of culinary possibilities. This adaptable ingredient may take your cuisine to new levels in both beverages and desserts, making every meal a pleasurable sensory experience. So explore the culinary possibilities of peppermint oil and discover the beauty of mint in your kitchen.

Using Peppermint Oil In Daily Life

One of the most adaptable essential oils, peppermint oil is used in many facets of daily life. Here, we'll look at some of the many uses for this aromatic and energizing oil, including cleaning and refreshing, dental care, and insect control.

1. Natural Solutions For Pest Control With Peppermint Oil:

An environmentally responsible and natural substitute for chemical pest control techniques is peppermint oil. Because of its potent yet attractive scent, it is well-recognized for its capacity to keep rodents and insects away. Here's how you use peppermint oil to get rid of pests:

Repelling Insects: To repel ants, spiders, and mosquitoes, combine a few drops of peppermint oil with water and mist it about windows, doors, and other entry points.

Cotton balls dipped in peppermint oil can be used as a rodent repellent by placing them in rodent-inhabited locations. The potent aroma of peppermint frequently deters rodents and mice.

Flea Control: To make a flea-repelling spray, combine a few drops of peppermint oil with a carrier oil or add it directly to your pet's shampoo.

Peppermint oil is a great option for people looking for a more natural approach to pest management because it is a non-toxic and pleasant-smelling substitute for chemical insecticides.

2. Peppermint For Cleaning And Freshening:

Your cleaning regimen will benefit greatly from the inclusion of peppermint oil. It's a useful tool for keeping a clean and comfortable living area because of its antibacterial and refreshing qualities. Peppermint oil can be used in the following ways to freshen and clean:

All-Purpose Cleaner: Combine water, white vinegar, and a small amount of peppermint oil to make an all-purpose cleaning spray. This concoction leaves surfaces smelling fresh as well as cleans.

Deodorizer: To refresh the air while you clean, add a few drops of peppermint oil to your vacuum cleaner's bag or filter.

Toilet Bowl cleaning: For a safe and efficient natural toilet bowl cleaning, combine baking soda, citric acid, and a few drops of peppermint oil.

The antibacterial qualities of peppermint oil can help you keep your home smelling nice and fresh while also assisting you in maintaining a clean and hygienic atmosphere.

3. Peppermint Oil In Dental Care:

Because peppermint oil naturally freshens breath and encourages good oral hygiene, it is a mainstay in dental care. It is frequently found in mouthwash, toothpaste, and other dental products. This is how dental care is improved with peppermint oil:

Fresh Breath: Peppermint oil's flavor and aroma can help fight bad breath and leave your mouth feeling revitalized.

Anti-Bacterial Properties: The natural antibacterial qualities of peppermint oil can help reduce the incidence of gum disease and cavities by controlling dangerous bacteria in the mouth.

Toothache Relief: For short-term relief from toothaches and oral discomfort, apply diluted peppermint oil to the affected area.

The benefits of peppermint oil for dental health go beyond mouth refreshing. Because of its natural qualities, it can promote general oral health and is therefore an important part of regular dental hygiene practices.

Peppermint oil has many uses in daily life, ranging from cleaning and pest control to dental care. Because of its adaptability and inherent qualities, it is a preferred option for people looking for non-toxic, sustainable solutions for a variety of everyday problems.

Warnings And Points To Take

The popular essential oil peppermint has many applications and advantages. To ensure safety and efficacy, peppermint oil should be used with caution and thought, just like any other strong substance. The following are important warnings and things to think about when using peppermint oil:

Take These Safety Measures Before Using Peppermint Oil:

1. Dilution: Because peppermint oil is so potent, applying it straight onto the skin may cause skin irritation. Before using it on the skin, always dilute it with a carrier oil, like jojoba or coconut oil. Usually, 1-2 drops of peppermint oil are diluted with one teaspoon of carrier oil.

2. Before applying peppermint oil topically, test a small area of your skin with a patch to see if you have any allergies or unpleasant effects.

This is particularly crucial if your skin is sensitive.

3. Steer clear of Contact with Eyes and Mucous Membranes: Peppermint oil can burn intensely if it gets in your eyes or on your mucous membranes. Use caution if you use it near your face, and properly wash your hands after using it.

4. Use Caution When Orally: Although extremely small amounts of peppermint oil can be consumed, care should be taken. Before consuming peppermint oil, you should always speak with a healthcare provider, particularly if you have any underlying medical conditions or are

currently taking medication. Because of its strength, the oil should never be taken in large amounts.

Sensitive Groups, Allergies, And Interactions:

1. Allergies: Peppermint oil may cause allergies in certain people. Consider getting an allergy test before using peppermint oil if you have a history of allergies to plants in the Lamiaceae family, which includes basil, lavender, and oregano.

2. Drug Interactions: Certain drugs, notably those that impact the liver, including cyclosporine and several

blood pressure medications, may interact with peppermint oil. If you take any prescription drugs, speak with your doctor to be sure there aren't any possible interactions.

3. Sensitive Groups: When taken as prescribed, peppermint oil is usually safe for adult use. However, it should not be given to newborns as it can be too strong for them. Additionally, women who are nursing or pregnant should use peppermint oil with caution and should first speak with a healthcare provider.

Dose:

1. Aromatherapy: To help with headaches, enhance mental clarity,

and lessen nausea, peppermint oil is frequently used in aromatherapy. To distribute the oil throughout the air, use a diffuser.

2. Topical Use: Dilute peppermint oil with a carrier oil before applying it topically to the skin to ease tension and aches in the muscles or to create a cooling effect.

3. Inhalation: The scent of peppermint oil is beneficial for clearing congestion and respiratory problems. You can inhale it straight from the bottle or create steam inhalation by adding a few drops to a bowl of hot water.

Avoids:

1. Take big Amounts: Peppermint oil can be poisonous, so never take big amounts of it. If you want to use it medicinally, stay with tiny, regulated doses and speak with a healthcare provider.

2. Use on Broken Skin: Since peppermint oil might aggravate already damaged skin, it is best not to apply it there.

3. Use on Pets: Pets may be poisoned by peppermint oil. Before using it near animals, keep it out of their reach and get advice from a veterinarian.

You may take advantage of peppermint oil's benefits while lowering the possibility of negative side effects and guaranteeing safe consumption according to these safety guidelines and considerations. If you have any questions or concerns about using peppermint oil, always get medical advice. This is especially important if you belong to a sensitive group or have underlying health issues.

Conclusion

A beneficial and adaptable essential oil, peppermint oil has many uses and advantages for a variety of areas of life. Peppermint oil has shown itself to be a beneficial addition to anyone's lifestyle, from its many health benefits to its useful applications in everyday tasks.

The adaptability of peppermint oil is one of its most amazing features. It can be used in aromatherapy to help calm the mind, induce relaxation, and reduce tension. For people seeking emotional balance and well-being, peppermint oil is a great option because of its energizing and refreshing aroma, which can instantly improve mood.

It's easy and satisfying to incorporate peppermint oil into your daily routine.

In terms of personal hygiene, it can be applied to ease headaches, release tense muscles, and ease gastrointestinal pain. It is a go-to remedy for many common illnesses due to its calming and cooling qualities. It is also used in dental hygiene products to support healthy gums and freshen breath.

In the kitchen, peppermint oil excels as well because it may give dishes a nice flavor boost. Peppermint oil adds a unique and energizing flavor to a variety of recipes, whether it is used in drinks, desserts, or savory dishes.

The advantages of peppermint oil also include its ability to repel pests, making it a healthy substitute for synthetic insecticides. Its potent scent can soothe itching bug bites and keep unpleasant pests out of your home.

Including peppermint oil in your daily regimen is not only sensible but also cost-effective. It's an affordable complement to your lifestyle because a little goes a long way. With its adaptability, you may use it for pest control, cooking excursions, aromatherapy, and personal care, all while getting the most out of your investment.

Finally, because peppermint oil has so many uses, it's a necessity to incorporate it into your daily routine.

Its many advantages, pleasant aroma, affordability, and convenience of use make it an invaluable tool that can improve your everyday routines and general well-being. Peppermint oil is a multipurpose and indispensable ally, whether your goal is to soothe, revitalize, or relieve tension.